Living & Thriving With Multiple Sclerosis

Sylvia Klineova, MD
Michelle Fabian, MD

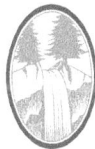

PROVENIR PUBLISHING

Spokane, Washington

www.provenirpublishing.com

Living And Thriving With Multiple Sclerosis

The authors, editors, and publisher have made every effort to provide accurate information. How-ever, they are not responsible for errors, omissions, or for any outcomes related to the use of contents of this book and take no responsibility for the use of the products and procedures described. The editors, editorial board, sponsoring organization, and publisher do not assume responsibility for the statements expressed by the authors in their contributions. Treatments and side effects described in this book may not be applicable to all people; likewise, some people may require a different treatment than described herein due to individual circumstances. Drugs and medical devices are discussed, but may have limited availability controlled by the Food and Drug Administration (FDA) for use only in a research study or clinical trial. Research, clinical practice, and government relations often change the accepted standard in the field. When consideration is being given to use of any drug in a clinical setting, the health care provider or reader is responsible for determining the optimal treatment for an individual patient and is responsible for reviewing the most up-to-date recommendations on dose, precautions, and contra indications, and determining the appropriate usage for the product. This is especially important in the case of drugs that are new or seldom used.

Published by Provenir Publishing, LLC, P. O. Box 211, Greenacres, WA 99016-0211

Production Credits

Lead Editor: Sylvia Klineova

Editors: Christopher Lee & Elizabeth Hanson

Art Director and Illustration: Micah Harman

Cover Design: Micah Harman

Printing History: August 2014, First Edition.

Contents

Introduction

If you (or somebody close to you) have just been diagnosed with multiple sclerosis (MS), you likely have many questions and might feel like you are not getting the answers you need. Perhaps the answers are confusing or maybe you don't understand the technical language of your doctor. This is potentially a challenging time for you: MS symptoms can be confusing and you will likely need some guidance.

The primary goal of this book is to help you understand what multiple sclerosis (MS) is, what causes it, what the potential associated problems are, and what to expect from medications used for treatment. This book is designed to offer you guidance in easily understandable language thus empowering you with knowledge for this journey.

Part One

What Is Multiple Sclerosis?

Multiple sclerosis, or MS, is a disease of the brain and spinal cord. Imagine that nerve cells and their endings function like electrical cables with sheets of insulation around them. These sheets of insulation are called "myelin". In someone with multiple sclerosis, myelin is destroyed from time to time by "inflammation".

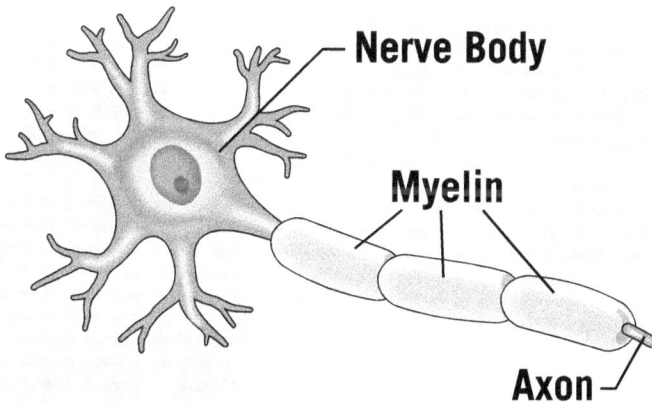

A Nerve cell and myelin sheath.

Inflammation is caused by normal blood cells (T and B cells) which are responsible for immunity. These cells protect us from bacteria, viruses, cancer cells, and other harmful organisms by attacking and destroy any potentially dangerous intruder. Under normal circumstances this is an important and beneficial process, but in people with multiple sclerosis those same immune cells attack and destroy myelin. Currently, there is no scientific explanation why this happens to some people and not others and who are at greatest risk.

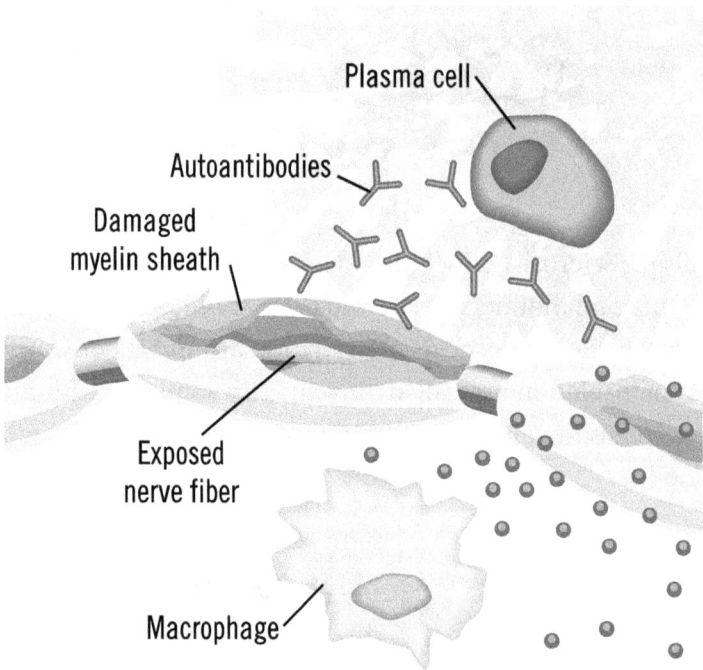

Damage to the myelin covering is caused by immune cells acting abnormally.

The destruction of myelin by inflammation is called "demyelination". Just as an electrical cable without insulation does not function properly, when myelin is lost or damaged, nerve cells are not able to send or carry information at the proper speed, and sometimes not at all. Myelin is also an important source of nourishment for nerve cells and endings. The loss of the myelin means the loss of nourishment which can lead to further nerve cell damage. Therefore, it is crucial to limit harmful demyelination.

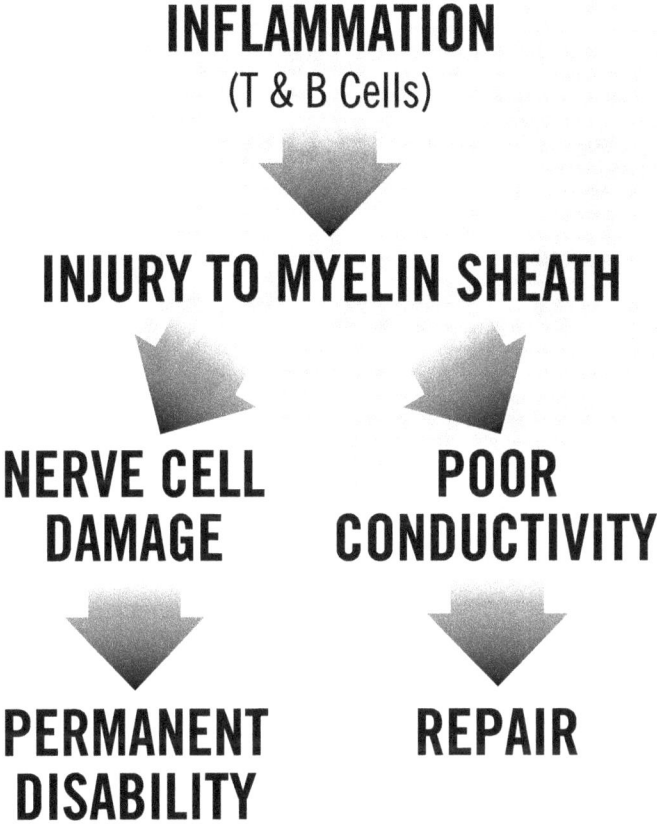

INFLAMMATION
(T & B Cells)

INJURY TO MYELIN SHEATH

NERVE CELL DAMAGE

POOR CONDUCTIVITY

PERMANENT DISABILITY

REPAIR

Demyelination process: Inflammation leads to myelin injury then, under normal circumstances, repair.

After a period of demyelination, the body is usually able to repair and replace the lost myelin: nerve cells regain their normal, or near normal, function. However, without treatment, demyelination goes unchecked and the body's ability to repair decreases while the possibility of permanent damage and impaired function increases.

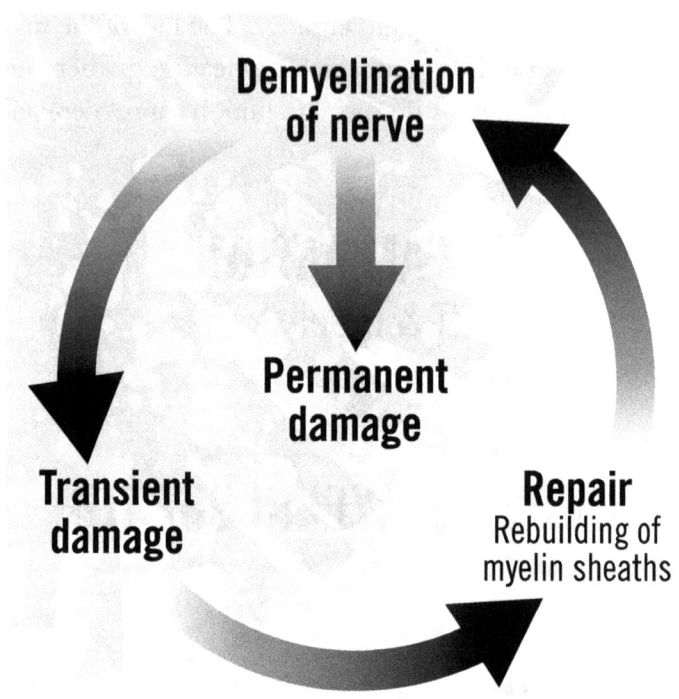

Demyelination can lead to temporary or permanent nerve injury.

Part Two

What Are The Common Symptoms Of Multiple Sclerosis?

There are many signs and symptoms of multiple sclerosis. "Symptoms" are based on the patient's own perception of feeling "differently". "Signs"are the abnormalities a doctor or caregiver finds during a physical examination. While "symptoms" and "signs" can be different for each person, a doctor would expect them to last more than 24 hours if they are caused by MS. The process of demyelination and migration of immune cells into the brain takes at least 24 hours so if a symptom or sign resolves within 24 hours, it is likely not caused by MS.

Key Point:

Symptoms and signs of multiple sclerosis are expected to last at least 24 hours.

The most common symptoms and signs caused by multiple sclerosis are:

Optic Neuritis (inflammation of the optic nerve) symptoms include loss of or blurred vision, usually in one eye, accompanied by some degree of pain associated with eye movement. Blurred vision can be very subtle, as if looking through clouded glass. A change in color vision is possible as well. Red is most commonly affected, but other colors can be affected. When viewing pictures, they often look "washed out". Symptoms are reversible for a majority of patients with vision returning back to normal within a couple of weeks to a few months.

Numbness and *tingling* can affect any part of the body and can spread over time. While not every occurrence of numbness affects a patient's ability to perform daily activities, it can cause problems with balance and walking (by making it difficult to recognize different surfaces). It is also quite common to feel an increased perception of touch, pain, itching, or electrical current running through the skin.

Patients may notice *muscle weakness* in the arms or legs causing slight weakness of the hand or foot, making everyday tasks challenging. They may also notice walking getting progressively difficult and their legs beginning to "drag". More pronounced loss of strength creates obvious impairments that are easily identifiable.

Frequent *balance problems* can cause periods when patients feel that either they, or the room, are "spinning". This limits their ability to walk and causes nausea and vomiting. Ringing in the ears or hearing loss are rare but can also occur in MS patients.

Frequent *Bowel* and *bladder problems* are common. Some patients experience constipation while others have diarrhea. Urgency and increased frequency of urination can be mixed with problems starting urination. A doctor will ask about losing bladder and bowel control and whether it is necessary to schedule activities within a close proximity to restrooms. Although loss of bowel and bladder control can be difficult to admit and discuss, doing so will help doctors make the correct diagnosis.

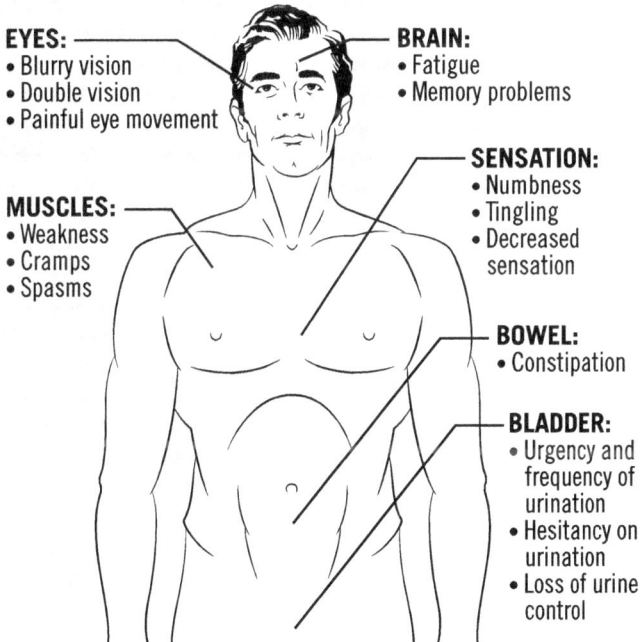

EYES:
• Blurry vision
• Double vision
• Painful eye movement

BRAIN:
• Fatigue
• Memory problems

SENSATION:
• Numbness
• Tingling
• Decreased sensation

MUSCLES:
• Weakness
• Cramps
• Spasms

BOWEL:
• Constipation

BLADDER:
• Urgency and frequency of urination
• Hesitancy on urination
• Loss of urine control

Main symptoms of multiple sclerosis.

Part Three

Common Causes Of Multiple Sclerosis

Although frustrating, the fact is physicians and scientists do not currently know, precisely, all of the causes of MS. What is known is that MS is a complex and variable disease.

An MS patient's immune system plays a leading role in the destruction of myelin and injury to the nerve cells, but it is not known what "triggers" this process and what perpetuates it. The manifestation of multiple sclerosis can be very different from patient to patient. This suggests that there are likely multiple triggers. Although several causes of multiple sclerosis are being studied, the leading ones are:

- *Genetic pre-disposition* or inclination to develop autoimmune diseases like multiple sclerosis.

- *Problems with regulation* of one's own immunity.

- *Environmental factors* such as exposure to viruses, especially Epstein-Barr virus.

- *Smoking* and *vitamin D* deficiency.

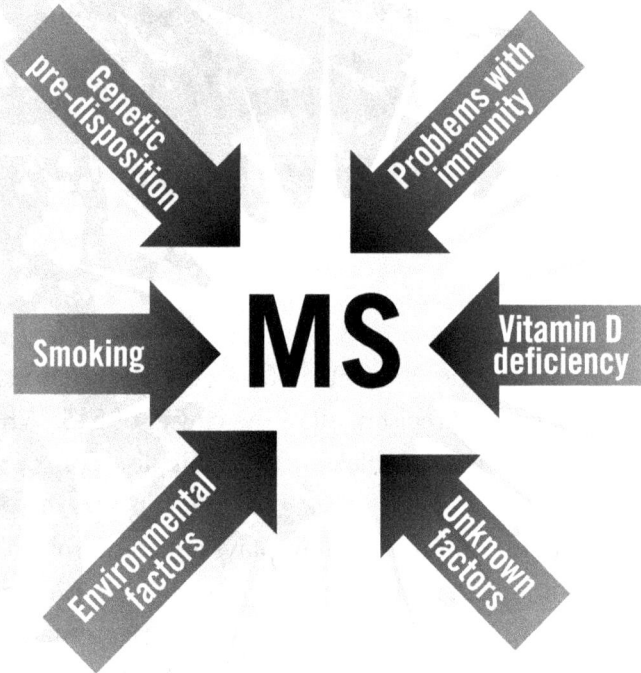

Proposed causes of multiple sclerosis.

Part Four

Standard Tests For Diagnosis

Diagnosing MS can be a complex task. There is no single testing method that can detect or eliminate the presence of MS. Currently, there is no blood or imaging test that can make a definitive diagnosis. Therefore, the diagnosis is made by combining a patient's history of clinical changes, a neurological examination, and the results from imaging studies (MRI) and laboratory tests. Using imaging studies as an additional diagnostic tool helps clinicians make a quicker diagnosis.

Diagnosis In The Past And Now

In the past, an MS diagnosis relied on the presence of two events of neurological impairment that affected two separate systems in the body, such as strength and ability to feel touch. These events also had to be separated by at least 30 days. Diagnosing MS in this way took a very long time, as these events could be separated by years. With the advancements of MRI techniques, clinicians are now able to combine history and MRI images to monitor symptoms and signs over a period of time.

Initial Interview

The MS diagnosis process starts with an interview by a neurologist followed by a neurological examination. During the interview a patient will be asked to describe, in chronological order, any neurological problems they have experienced in the past. The most common type of multiple sclerosis (relapsing–remitting MS or RRMS) presents itself in a pattern of disease activity (relapse) and disease rest (remission). As previously mentioned, symptoms and signs must last longer than 24 hours to be considered a relapse. It is important to know whether the onset of symptoms was sudden or gradual and whether relapse symptoms resolved completely, partially, or continued to worsen. Establishing this pattern by using a detailed history and time periods is crucial for the diagnosis.

Neurological Examination

The neurological exam is an important part of diagnosis. During the exam, the doctor will be able to identify any impairment that the disease might have caused (some of which the patient might not be aware). The patient's cooperation and effort will be the key to a successful, objective exam.

The neurological exam consists of testing various parts of the nervous system including vision, strength and function of various muscles, and the ability to feel different sensations (light touch, sharp touch, vibration, and temperature). Balance and fine hand movements are tested as well as a patient's ability and time needed to walk 25 feet. This is a common measure used to evaluate subtle changes in strength, balance, and speed. In addition, a patient might be asked to walk on heels and toes, and walk heal to toe in a straight line. This helps the doctor discern any subtle changes in walking ability and balance.

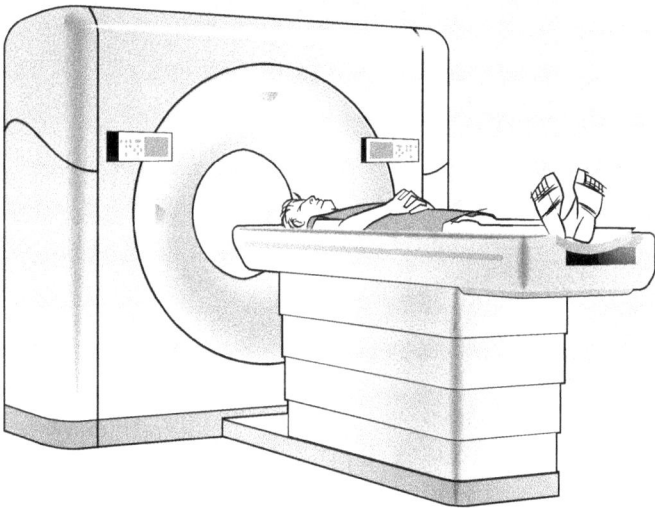

MRI scanners are utilized to obtain detailed brain images and assist in the diagnosis of multiple sclerosis.

Imaging Tests

Imaging tests are a vital part of the diagnosis and monitoring of MS. **Magnetic Resonance Imaging** (MRI) is widely used today to improve a doctor's ability to diagnose MS earlier and more accurately.

MRI uses a large magnetic field and radio waves to produce highly detailed images of the brain and spinal cord. It is a painless procedure that requires the patient to lie still within the enclosed magnetic field of the imaging device. MRI's are known for the loud noise that is produced during the exam. This noise is perfectly normal. Open MRI scanners are available, but are not preferred because they usually produce lower quality images. Some imaging centers cancel the noise and reduce distractions by playing music through headphones worn by the patient. Imaging for diagnosis and monitoring of MS takes about an hour and requires IV contrast dye. IV contrast dye is a liquid agent, injected through a small catheter in the forearm vein, used for assessing activity of the disease. Unless the patient is allergic to the dye, the contrast agent is rarely harmful. If kidney function is decreased, the contrast dye cannot be used. Depending on the patient's age and medical history, simple blood tests might be done before an MRI test.

MRI produces highly detailed images of the brain and spinal cord. In MS patients, MRI shows noticeable white spots commonly called "lesions" or "plaques". Other diseases can produce white spots on MRI, but only lesions with a specific appearance in specific locations are caused by MS. New, active MS lesions absorb the contrast agent creating a shining or "lit-up" appearance called "enhancement" on the MRI image. Enhancement lasts for 1-3 months after which the immune cells stop their destruction and the lesion "quiets down" and forms a scar. At that point, contrast dye will not absorb into the lesion and although the lesion is still visible on MRI images, it will not "light up".

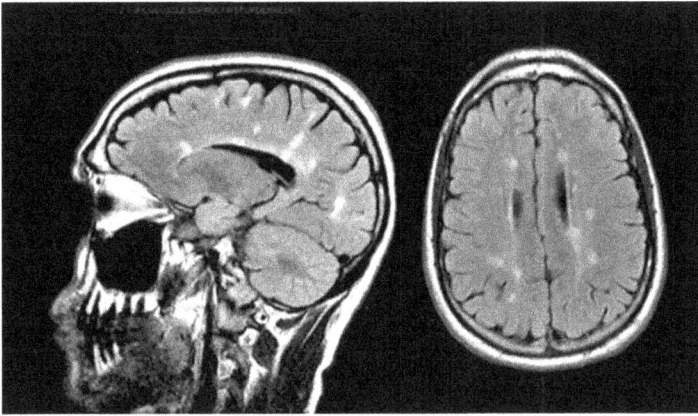

The frequency of MRI imaging can vary according to physician preference, but patients can generally expect to have an MRI of the brain and spine done at the time of diagnosis and when new symptoms indicating a relapse appear. It is common to have a yearly MRI to help doctors monitor the disease and look for active inflammation (a sign of ongoing disease). It is not unusual for patients to have new lesions visible on MRI without any new noticeable symptoms. These are called "silent lesions".

Spinal Tap

Another procedure used for diagnosis is a spinal tap. This procedure is used to sample the cerebrospinal fluid that surrounds the brain and spinal cord and test it for the presence of proteins called **oligoclonal bands**. While the majority of patients with MS have these diagnostic proteins present, there are some patients without them.

In a spinal tap, a needle is placed in the space between the bones of the spinal canal and fluid is removed for testing. In some ways, it is similar receiving epidural anesthesia during childbirth. During the procedure, the patient is placed in a sitting or lying position with their chin on their chest. Remaining still and in the correct position during the procedure are necessary for a successful spinal tap. Local anesthetics are used to diminish pain but one will feel pressure when the spinal needle is inserted and the fluid is drawn.

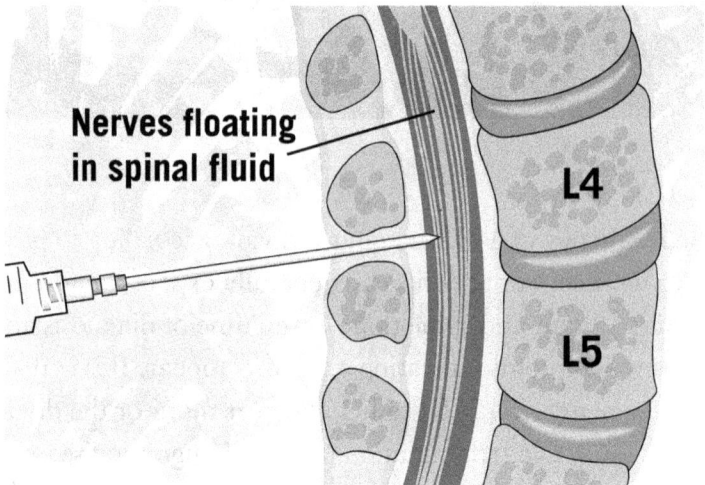

A needle is placed in the spinal canal to test for multiple sclerosis by measuring proteins.

After the spinal tap the patient is monitored for a brief period. If there are no complications the patient can return home. Physicians might choose to do this test in their office or, in some circumstances, will refer the patient to a radiologist so the procedure can be done under X-ray guidance. Headache or slight pain in the lower back can be experienced after a spinal tap. Headache is caused by a change in pressure resulting from the fluid removal. It will commonly increase while standing and quickly improve while lying down. This is uncomfortable but not dangerous and usually resolves after a few days' rest. Drinking caffeinated beverages can help relieve headache as well.

Blood Tests

Blood tests are a routine part of the diagnostic process. However, they are usually used to test for, and eliminate, diseases that manifest in a manner similar to MS. The most common tests are thyroid function, vitamin B12, and folate levels. Rheumatologic conditions, such as lupus, Sjogren's syndrome, and others are tested as well.

Vitamin D

The role of vitamin D in multiple sclerosis is being studied but no conclusive results have been established. Vitamin D deficiency can contribute to developing MS, but it is not certain how the level of vitamin D can affect patients who already have MS. Nevertheless, it is common among MS specialists to test vitamin D levels and use supplements in order to maintain high-normal levels.

Part Five

Severity: Graded Or Measured

Multiple sclerosis can be divided into subtypes based on how MS develops and runs its course. Medical research and discovery continue to reveal new and useful information which will likely result in changes to the subtype classifications in the future. This book will define and discuss three common subtypes of MS.

Relapsing And Remitting MS Subtype

About 85% of patients, have **relapsing–remitting MS** (RRMS). RRMS is characterized by periods of "relapse" (disease activity) and periods of "remission" (disease inactivity). During relapse, one experiences certain neurological problems or symptoms; most likely blurred and/or double vision, painful eye movement, weakness, numbness, tingling, or feeling of electric current running through the spine when bending the head forward. A patient might also experience balance problems or worsening of fine motor skills. These problems usually start gradually, worsen during the next couple of days, and will always last more than 24 hours. The symptoms usually subside, gradually, over a couple of days or weeks (this can happen with or without any treatment).

During periods of remission, patients might continue to experience brief ongoing symptoms; occasional numbness, tingling, and imbalance. But generally speaking, during remission, symptoms are stable and don't change dramatically. Periods of remission can last several years and are the ultimate goal of the treatments. New relapses cause either a completely new neurological symptom or significant worsening of an existing symptom. Relapse is considered "new" if it happens more than 30 days after the previous relapse.

Secondary Progressive MS Subtype

The second subtype of MS is called **secondary progressive MS** (SPMS). It is characterized by a slow, gradual progression, usually occurring after years of relapsing-remitting disease. In this case, the patient notices a slow and gradual increase in severity of ongoing symptoms, such as increased weakness, more balance problems, greater difficulty walking, and a need for a cane or walker. This slow progression might not be noticeable at first because symptoms can fluctuate over short periods of time. It is best to evaluate worsening symptoms over the previous 6 months to a year.

Doctors evaluate a patient's neurological status using real life scenarios such as using landmarks (like city blocks)to evaluate how far a patient is able to walk and whether there is a change. Another sign of progression is an increased need for assistance (i.e. exchanging a cane for a walker or using assistance consistently). Exercise intolerance and stopping gym visits, though subtle, should be reported to a doctor.

While there are no approved treatments currently available for this subtype of MS, there are interventions and health changes that can increase the quality of life substantially. If care is established at a comprehensive center, clinical studies may also be available to patients with this subtype.

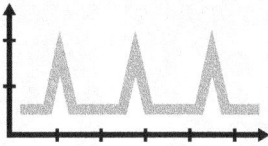

RRMS
Relapsing Remitting MS

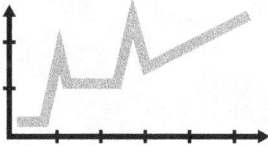

SPMS
Secondary Progressive MS

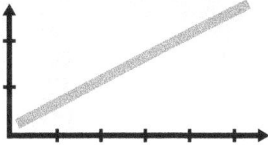

PPMS
Primary Progressive MS

Types of multiple sclerosis.

Primary Progressive MS Subtype

Primary progressive MS (PPMS) is the third subtype of MS. PPMS progresses over time with no clear periods of relapses. Despite its name, PPMS progression can be slow and can reach a steady state with stable neurological status. However, disability does increase over time.

Multiple sclerosis symptoms vary for each patient. Some people can be impaired by early disability, but the majority of patients continue their lives with minimal symptoms and thrive. There is no single measure for disease severity, rather a tendency to use variable measures and terms.

Typically, disease severity is measured using changes in MRI results, development of new relapses, and evidence of progressive symptoms. More frequent relapses mean higher disease activity and usually more severe symptoms. In progressive types of multiple sclerosis, severity can be judged by how fast the progression of disability happens.

MRI provides another measure of the severity of the disease. The number of lesions, also called "lesion load", is used as an indicator of severity. The amount of lesions visible on MRI images is called the "disease burden". While an exact number is often difficult to estimate, the terms: low, moderate, or high lesion load or disease burden are used. Active inflammation, visible on MRI scans as an abnormal area, is another way disease activity is judged.

The presence of enhancing lesions can be used to estimate the activity level of the disease process. More frequent inflammation means higher activity of the disease.

Some physicians use "benign" or "malignant" MS in an attempt to characterize disease situations. Benign characterizing very low or insignificant disability and malignant characterizing significant neurological impairment, such as dependency on walking aids or help of others. While a "benign" characterization suggests a better course of the disease, it should not be misinterpreted to mean that medications or treatment are not necessary. Multiple sclerosis is an unpredictable disease and can lead to different types of impairment later in life.

Part Six

Treatment Team

Multiple sclerosis treatments have evolved and become more complex over the last twenty years. Today, treatment requires a team of experts in their field rather than a single person providing care to patients).

MS specialists (neurologists with additional training exclusively in MS) typically lead the care team. Specialists are trained in the latest research and care guidelines. Unfortunately, these specialists are usually only available in major cities or university hospital settings. Travel distance can often be a daunting challenge for patients desiring care from a specialist.

In most cases, general neurologists are qualified to provide care to patients. However, with more sophisticated treatments becoming available, general neurologists might find it challenging to stay current and/or adapt. Many patients see a specialist once or twice a year and see their general neurologist for regular visits or in case of an emergency.

If MS care is provided in a comprehensive center, patients

will typically meet various other people during their visits. Teaching or university hospitals provide education to neurology fellows who are training to become specialists in multiple sclerosis. At these centers, it is probable that one or two fellows will attend visits along with a patient's regular MS doctor.

Some centers also work closely with psychiatrists or psychologists who are available to help when needed. Referring a patient to a psychiatrist with a specific knowledge of multiple sclerosis significantly enhances the care that patient receives.

Other physicians, in different medical specialties, are commonly part of the team. Ophthalmologists (or neuro-ophthalmologists) and urologists are often needed to provide care for health concerns (i.e. vision and bladder problems) associated with MS. In some cases one visit may be all that is needed but when more care is necessary, a patient will continue regular visits.

A patient's initial phone contact might be with a nurse practitioner. Nurse practitioners (highly trained and specialized nurses) at most of the MS centers are supervised by, and work closely with, doctors but tend to their patients independently. They are an indispensable part of the team and bring additional focused expertise to health care.

Physical and occupational therapists, together with physiatrists, may also be part of a patient's care team. Physical therapy and exercise, under proper supervision, can be helpful; often leading to a better quality of life. Patients might need physical therapy only a few times during the course of their MS, but they might also find regular sessions helpful in retaining strength and stamina.

Social workers are also an invaluable support to a comprehensive center. They provide help guiding patients toward community support, disability applications, and transportation solutions. Their primary goal is to make sure that a patient's well-being is sustained and they never feel alone or stranded.

Research is a major focus at university hospitals and care centers. If a patient chooses to participate in any research project, they will meet with research coordinators during their visits. Research coordinators make sure that every project runs smoothly and patients are protected and safe during participation. By taking part in a research project, patients can be part of exciting future discoveries in multiple sclerosis.

Part Seven

Treatments And Side Effects: Choosing Treatment

Recent research has provided much needed development to MS therapies. Doctors can now offer a wide array of FDA approved medications to patients. The primary goal of these therapies is to reduce the disease activity to a minimum and prevent further impairment. Before starting any treatment, patients should understand that the treatments used are not typically able to resolve previous symptoms and impairments. Those often remain unchanged or improve on their own with time.

The majority of medications used are "**preventative medications**". The goal of preventative medications is to prevent further relapses and the occurrence of silent lesions on MRI.

Because the disease differs in each patient, this goal is met in varying degrees. To determine the effectiveness of a particular medication, a doctor will consider the number of relapses and the MRI activity together. It is never a black or white decision and can take time.

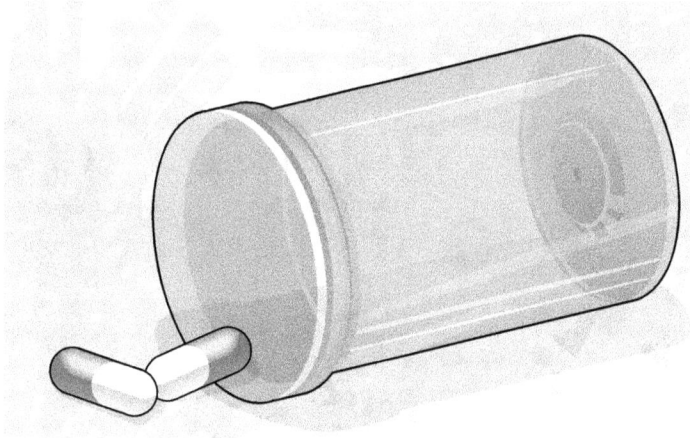

The treatments for multiple sclerosis have evolved significantly in recent years.

There are two main groups of treatment in multiple sclerosis: **treatments for acute relapses** and **preventative disease modifying treatments**, or **DMT**s.

Acute relapses are usually treated with steroids. The goal of this treatment is to stop acute inflammation. Steroids do not treat the MS itself, but shorten the time of relapse symptoms in a patient. It is similar to giving acetaminophen for a fever and cold symptoms. Although the acetaminophen is not treating the cold, it is working to shorten the duration and lessen the symptoms. It is important to understand that with or without steroids, the relapse will eventually end. Permanent leftover effects from the relapse are not influenced by steroids. However, a relapse may be shorter and less severe with steroids. In other words, steroids get the symptoms "better *quicker*", but not "better *better*". Thus, doctors may choose to treat a relapse with steroids when a patient is experiencing trouble with vision, walking, or pain, but may not give steroids if the relapse is not particularly bothersome.

Steroids can be given in the form of pills: a course lasting up to 10 days. More often, patients will receive steroids in the form of an IV infusion through a small catheter. This treatment is given daily for about an hour and can last from 3 to 5 days. Some improvement of symptoms can be seen while receiving the treatment, but effects can be lasting and improvement continues many weeks or months afterwards. While taking steroids, patients are directed to take over-the-counter medications for stomach protection. Steroids can also increase appetite and thirst, raise blood sugar level, and can cause dramatic mood changes. Typically the risk of these side effects is low, but those with high blood pressure or diabetes should inform their doctor. Infusions are given either in a doctor's office, the infusion center at the hospital, or during hospital stays. Sometimes hospital stays are necessary for patients with additional diseases and those unable to walk and/or take care of themselves.

The second group of medications is called **disease-modifying therapies** (DMTs). DMTs are used to prevent further relapses and disease activity. Recent developments have brought many new medications to the market.

Injectable medications have been available for over twenty years. The two most common injectable agents are **interferons** and **glatiramer acetate**. Both work by shifting immune system activity gently away from attacking nerve cells and toward protecting them. Because of this gentle shift, patients are not prone to an increased rate of infections.

All of the **interferons** are injected under the skin or into the muscle; a simple procedure the patient will be taught (usually by a nurse practitioner). Frequency of injections can vary from once a week to every other day.

Common side effects of interferons are flu-like symptoms: shakes, slight fever, muscle ache, and headache. Symptoms usually start a couple of hours after the injection and usually respond to treatment with acetaminophen or ibuprofen. Side effects from long-term use are worsening liver function and mood changes (making patients more prone to depression). While on interferons, liver function and blood cell count should be monitored every three months. Patients should report any significant mood changes that occur.

Glatiramer acetate is injected under the skin every day or three times a week. It usually has a very low occurrence of side effects but can cause pain at injection sites or skin changes with long-term use. There are no blood tests required while using glatiramer acetate.

For any injectable medication used, the correct technique and rotating of injection sites is recommended to prevent pain and skin changes. Even patients who have been injecting themselves for an extended time can benefit from re-training.

Another medication used more widely today is **natalizumab**. Available since 2004, natalizumab prevents immune cells from entering the brain and, in this way, protects patients from new disease attacks.

Natalizumab is given by an IV infusion at a specialized infusion center every 28 days. This treatment procedure usually takes up to three hours and, after brief monitoring, the patient is safe to go home. Natalizumab is a safe and well tolerated medication without significant side effects. The primary risk associated with this therapy is a brain infection (occurring under specific circumstances) called PML. PML is caused by JC virus, carried by about 50% of the population. Ordinarily, this virus lives undetected in the body without causing any symptoms or problems; natalizumab can increase the risk of activating the JC virus causing PML. Before considering natalizumab as suitable therapy, antibodies to JC virus have to be evaluated with a simple blood test. For those with a negative test (no previous JC virus infection), this medication might be a good option. If the test is positive, consideration of natalizumab requires a careful discussion about the risks this treatment might pose. While taking natalizumab, liver function tests and blood cell counts should be checked every three months and JC virus antibodies every six months.

Oral medications are the newest treatments; available since 2010. Currently, there are three types of pills: differing in their mechanism of action, frequency of doses, and side effects.

Fingolimod is the oldest oral medication approved for treatment (since 2010). It is a pill taken once a day and is usually well tolerated. Fingolimod traps certain types of immune cells in lymph nodes (the usual home for immune cells) and prevents them from travelling in the blood stream toward the brain. However, it does not increase a patient's susceptibility to infection.

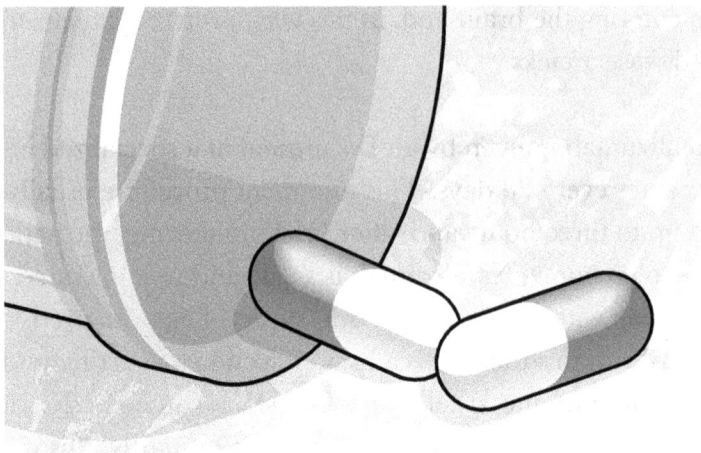

There are multiple oral medications available for treatment of multiple sclerosis.

There are heart and eye risks and side effects associated with fingolimod. In some patients, within 24 hours of the first dose, fingolimod can cause a slow heart rate and low blood pressure. An evaluation by a cardiologist or internist and an ECG are required before starting the treatment. It also requires monitoring (frequent checks of blood pressure and pulse) for 6 hours after the first dose. This monitoring is done in clinics specifically equipped and attended by the proper staff to handle any complications. Eye doctors should regularly evaluate the drug's effect on the eyes every three to six months during the treatment. Testing liver function and blood cell counts should also be done every three months.

Teriflunomide has been approved since September 2012, but it is not entirely a new medication. It is related to leflunomide, an agent used to treat rheumatoid arthritis. Taken once a day, this medication works by decreasing production of a certain portion of the immune cells that are thought to be responsible for attacking the patient's body. The immune cells responsible for protection against infection remain unaffected.

Side effects include nausea and abdominal pain, and a risk of worsening liver function. Less common side effects are hair thinning, vomiting, and diarrhea. Teriflunomide stays in the patient's body for an extended time; even after treatment has ended. When starting new treatments with different medication, a patient will have to undergo an elimination procedure to remove the residual teriflunomide from their system. This procedure involves taking another medication, commonly used for the treatment of high cholesterol, three times a day for 11 days. This agent, called "cholestyramine", will bind residual teriflunomide and remove it from the patient's body. Except for an unpleasant taste, cholestyramine poses no additional risks. Liver function tests and blood cell counts should be checked every month for the first six months and every three months afterwards.

BG-12 or **dimethyl fumarate** is the newest oral medication; available since March 2013. Like teriflunomide, it is not a completely new medication, but could be considered a "cousin" of treatment agents used in Germany for psoriasis. BG-12 works against inflammation, which is the cause of demyelination that can lead to MS.

Taken twice a day, BG-12 can cause stomach and intestinal related side effects. There is a possibility of nausea and vomiting, bloating, abdominal pain, and sometimes diarrhea at the outset of treatment. Most patients can lower the risk of these side effects by taking BG-12 with food. Another common harmless, but uncomfortable, side effect is skin flushing. After taking the medication, a patient's skin can turn red, warm, and sometimes itchy. Flushing usually lasts a short time; from a few minutes to a couple of hours. Again, taking medication with food can lower the risk of skin flushing.

Every medication has potential side effects. The severity of side effects can vary from patient to patient. It is also quite possible that no side effects will be experienced. Doctors will list all of the potential and reported side effects, but a patient should know that, while it is a risk, it is not a certainty that side effects will occur. Calm vigilance is always a good approach when monitoring side effects. Experiencing side effects, "out of the ordinary" in nature or severity, is always a good reason to call the doctor.

There are many medications to choose from. Choosing the right medication for an individual patient should be the result of a thorough discussion between patient and physician. While doctors will provide all of the necessary information and guidance, it is the patient taking the medication who will benefit from the treatment and experience its side effects. Making the optimal clinical decision requires considering multiple factors such as the disease course, its activity and severity, and lifestyle choices and preferences. While some patients prefer older, longer proven, and safe medications (despite injecting themselves), others will choose newer treatment agents because of oral administration. A physician's knowledge and guidance will play an important role, but the patient ultimately makes the decision. A patient should always ask about side effects, risks, and the frequency of monitoring that each medication requires. Understanding how a particular medication will change one's lifestyle is important. The patient should always be in agreement with a treatment decision.

Acquiring additional information can be beneficial to patients and their families, if the information is objective and based on facts. The internet can provide conflicting information and a patient's doctor should be able to point them toward the best resources. The National Multiple Sclerosis Society is an excellent source for information about the drugs currently used. Additionally, the web sites of individual companies manufacturing the medications provide more commercial, but accurate information. Joining online support or discussion groups can also be a good way to exchange information and ideas; understanding however, the ever-present risk of acquiring subjective experiences and thoughts. Patients should always be very careful about new treatments, ideas, or products and should always check with their physicians about the credibility of this information.

Part Eight

Symptomatic Treatment

Multiple sclerosis can cause many symptoms. It is important to remember that there are many ways to treat them and improve the quality of life. Taking a proactive approach in symptom management is the best way to get them under optimal control. This requires talking about each of the symptoms with a doctor to create a unique treatment plan.

Fatigue is the most common symptom reported by MS patients. Medications like interferons can cause fatigue, but patients treated with different agents, or not treated at all, can also experience fatigue. Since the precise cause of fatigue is not known, finding the right treatment is often challenging. The first step in evaluating MS-related fatigue is to rule out any other causes. Sleep problems, depression, pain, thyroid dysfunction, anemia, and medications are all causes of fatigue that should be considered. After excluding all other causes, treatment for fatigue should then be considered. The usual "rule of thumb" practiced by MS doctors is to try simple remedies before any medications are started. Physical exercise, improving sleep patterns, and decreasing workloads and stress are all interventions that can potentially decrease fatigue. If these are unsuccessful, there are a few medications that are helpful for many patients. The main side effects of these treatment agents include: increased agitation, nervousness, and low appetite.

Pain affects some, but not all, patients with MS. It can limit daily activity and reduce quality of life. There are two main sources of pain associated with MS; either **neuropathic** pain or **musculoskeletal** pain. Neuropathic pain, the most common source, is caused by damage to cells, nerve endings, and brain centers responsible for pain perception. Additionally, patients may have musculoskeletal pain (pain in muscles and joints). Musculoskeletal pain is not directly caused by MS, but by changes in walking as a result of weakness and spasticity which puts increased stress on the joints and muscles.

In many cases, medications used for the treatment of neuropathic pain were originally used for other diseases, such as epilepsy and depression. These medications are designed to alter brain chemicals. It can take time to find the right medication and dose to effectively control pain. Side effects of these medications are uncommon, but may include: sleepiness, weight gain, worsening of liver function, and changes in cell counts. Opioids (medications traditionally used for pain treatment) are rarely ideal for MS patients because their side effects (significant sedation, increased fatigue, and balance issues) exacerbate some MS symptoms. Musculoskeletal pain is best treated with anti-inflammatory agents as well as physical therapy.

Spasticity, muscle tightness causing cramps, spasms, or increased difficulty walking, is another common symptom of MS. The initial treatment of spasticity is stretching. Short sessions of stretching throughout the day (5 minutes 5 times a day) can offer significant relief. Additionally, anti-spasticity medications are available when stretching does not satisfactorily alleviate all of the symptoms. The main side effect of anti-spasticity medications is sedation. Doses are usually tailored to the patient's individual tolerance and symptom relief.

Increased urgency and frequency of urination is a common side effect significantly affecting quality of life. Planning life around bathroom breaks and waking multiple times during the night to urinate can take its toll on a patient's well-being. Discussing urinary habits or urinary problems with the neurologist can be embarrassing, but doing so can improve a patient's quality of life significantly. An MS physician might start treatment with a medication immediately, or may refer the patient to a urologist. The main side effects of medications used to treat urinary problems are: dry mouth, occasional blurry vision, and difficulty starting urination. If a patient has difficulty starting urination, they should stop the medication and call their doctor immediately.

Constipation, diarrhea, and bowel urgency (having to rush to the bathroom to make it in time) are common and should be discussed with a doctor. While medications for bowel symptoms are available over the counter in every pharmacy, changes in diet and lifestyle should be explored first. Registered dieticians, available in every major hospital, can help a patient change their dietary goals to determine the trigger of bowel problems. Increasing dietary fiber usually helps reduce bowel urgency and diarrhea, while dry fruits, prunes and prune juice help reduce constipation.

Remember that every medication used to treat additional symptoms caused by MS will have some side effects. Treatments should be tailored to the patient's needs and used when appropriate. If the side effects from the treatments reduce the quality of life, the treatments should be discontinued.

Part Nine

Lifestyle Recommendations

Often, patients want to take a "holistic" approach to treating their MS. The holistic approach, as defined by an MS specialist, is the appropriate MS treatment plus a healthy lifestyle. Healthy lifestyle choices can significantly improve the quality of life of an MS patient. It is important to maintain a healthy weight by eating foods that are nutritious: fruits and vegetables, with other foods, eaten in moderation, is a good diet to follow. As mentioned earlier, a registered dietician can help get one's diet on the right track. These days, it is common for patients to adopt a strict diet, such as gluten-free or dairy-free. It is likely that these diets are not dangerous, still MS specialists do not recommend them. There is no evidence that they are an effective treatment for MS. Similarly, there is no specific vitamin regimen that has been proven to treat MS. Vitamin D deficiency has been associated with increased risk of MS and possibly increased risk for MS progression. Although there is no current evidence that supplementing vitamin D will treat MS, most MS specialists agree that keeping the level of vitamin D in a normal range is a good idea.

Alcohol can be enjoyed in moderation, though some patients find their symptoms to temporarily worsen after having an alcoholic drink. In this case, especially if the symptoms are bothersome, alcohol should be avoided.

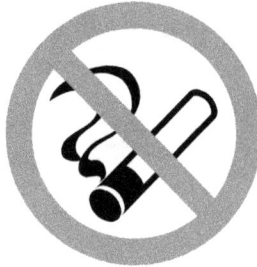

Smoking has also been associated with an increased risk of contracting MS. It has also been shown to increase the risk of a severe MS course. It is strongly suggested that an MS patient who smokes, quit.

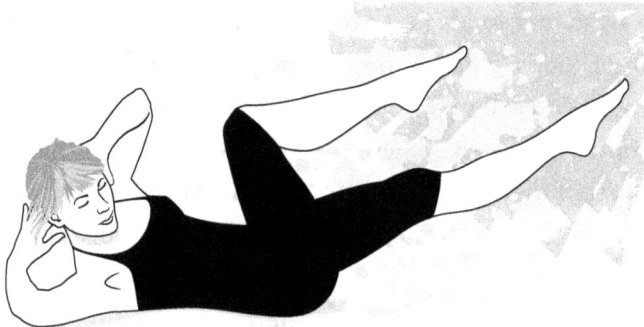

Exercise is especially important for MS patients. Not only does exercise strengthen the muscles, but it also helps patients with cognitive, as well as mood, symptoms. There is no specific exercise that is best for MS patients. It is important to choose an exercise routine that a patient likes to do or it is likely to be abandoned quickly.

Complementary treatments, such as acupuncture, meditation, and massage therapy are all safe treatments and improve the general quality and life for many MS patients.

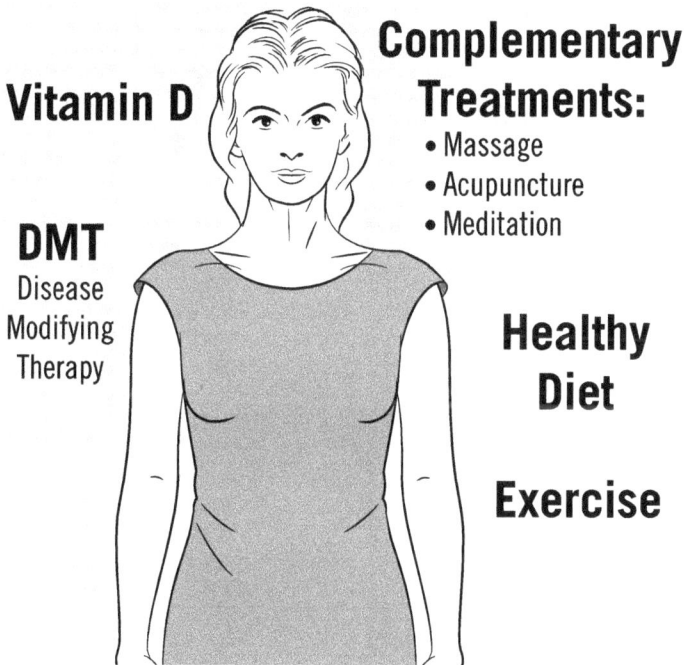

Vitamin D

Complementary Treatments:
• Massage
• Acupuncture
• Meditation

DMT
Disease Modifying Therapy

Healthy Diet

Exercise

Treatment approach for multiple sclerosis.

Notes

About The Authors

Sylvia Klineova, MD: Dr. Klineova is a practicing MS specialist and researcher at the Corinne Goldsmith Dickinson Center for MS at Mount Sinai (New York, NY). Dr. Klineova received her MD degree from P.J. Safarik University in Kosice, Slovakia and completed her residency at the Medical University of South Carolina. She joined CGD Center for MS as a Fellow in 2012. In addition to her clinical responsibilities at the CGD Center for MS, she is also Principal Investigator for clinical trials performed at the New York Eye and Ear Infirmary at Mount Sinai.

Michelle T. Fabian, MD: Dr. Fabian joined the Corinne Goldsmith Dickinson Center for MS as a Fellow in 2009. She completed her neurology residency at Mount Sinai Medical Center. A graduate of the University of Notre Dame, Dr. Fabian received her MD degree from Case Western Reserve University. In addition to her clinical responsibilities, she is currently Principal Investigator for multiple clinical trials performed at the CGD Center.

www.ingramcontent.com/pod-product-compliance
Lightning Source LLC
Chambersburg PA
CBHW060522280326
41933CB00014B/3071